# The Alkaline Diet Program:

*How to Reverse and Prevent Disease, Rejuvenate Your Body and Lose Weight Effectively, Plus 35 Great Recipes, Drinks and Shakes*

*By Juliette Sommers*

or implied. Readers acknowledge that the author is not engaging in the rendering of legal, financial, medical or professional advice.

By reading this document, the reader agrees that under no circumstances are we responsible for any losses, direct or indirect, which are incurred as a result of the use of information contained within this document, including, but not limited to; errors, omissions, or inaccuracies.

# Table of Contents

# Introduction

The Alkaline diet comes under several names, and they are all basically the same thing, essentially. The affirmed truth with this diet is that certain foods affect the acidity and PH levels of the body's fluids. Following this analysis, it is also proven in some research studies that this diet can be used to treat or prevent diseases. This is one of the reasons that the diet is mentioned throughout various clinical studies, incorporating the increased knowledge regarding the longevity of life and its expressed ability to aid in fending off illness and disease, from a nutrition stand point.

I will explain not only how the diet works, but also the long-term benefits of the Alkaline diet. As this diet is based on PH levels, it has been shown the PH body levels are affected by the mineral density of the foods you consume. The recommended PH level is around 7.5, which it is said can stop diseases and illnesses which are unable to thrive if the PH level of the body is within the recommended range. As your body PH level is a natural thing, this diet doesn't aim to change anything, its aim is just to get your body back on track and keep it at a more stable level.

*"Disease cannot live in an alkaline body"* Dr. Otto Warburg

# *Chapter 1: What is the Alkaline Diet?*

The Alkaline diet is a diet that helps to not only get your body's PH level back to where it should be, but to also maintain this in the long term. All living organisms and life forms depend on set PH levels, although, each organism has different levels compared to what the human body is. Your PH level changes depending on the foods that you eat. The meaning of PH is potential of hydrogen, and this is the measure of acidity or alkalinity of the body. Essentially, this is why if you eat a lot of food which is high in acids, your body goes into a state of acidosis - which is fundamentally an electrolyte imbalance.

The human body has a range of 7.3 to 7.4 on a balanced level with 7 being neutral, this is normally lower than what your body will be depending on what you eat or have eaten and the time of day. It is worth noting when acidity in the body raises the levels of minerals fall. So you could see a level of between 5 and 7, when acidity takes over.

Here I will explain how the diet works and some points of how the diet can be of benefit to you. It is believed since the cave man days to the present day, there have been changes in the acid load of the human diet. Due to food being mass industrialized over the last couple of hundred years, food crops now contain less chloride, magnesium, and potassium, with increased sodium.

It is the kidneys function to maintain the electrolyte levels so when you are exposed to over acidic foods, the electrolytes are used to counteract the acid buildup. With the changes in the way, food crops are processed and the average American consumes three times as much sodium as potassium. With the increase in sodium levels being consumed, there are also decreases in potassium, magnesium, fiber and antioxidants, so on top of all this, an average diet is very high in refined fats and sugars.

As a result, these changes mean that an average person's PH level is no longer at the optimal level, and this is coupled with a low nutrient intake especially magnesium and potassium. Effects on the body because of this are accelerated aging, a gradual loss of organ functions and lessened bone strength, which is the result of high acidity which steals minerals from the bones, cells, and tissues.

The complete PH level range is 0 – 14 with 7 being neutral and above 7 being called basic, so anything under 7 is acidic. There are many people who test their PH level by their urine, although this can be used as a guide, it is not totally reliable as this is the way the body flushes out the system so the levels may be interpreted incorrectly. Actually, the ideal way is to use litmus paper on the tongue. It is also worth noting that litmus paper is inexpensive and can be bought easily online. Some parts of the body are supposed to be acidic for the body to function - a good example of this is the stomach which is filled with acids which break down the foods we eat.

In the case of a person's blood falling out of the PH range, this can really be very serious, especially if it continues long term.

One subject which can be added, although not essentially a part of this diet is the use of Alkaline drinking water. Fundamentally, this does have a higher PH level than normal tap water which is classed as slightly acidic, and it is stated that the consumption of Alkaline water gives more nutrients and is more easily absorbed by the body. Additionally, at present there have not been enough studies conducted to prove that the use of Alkaline water does present any adverse health effects. If Alkaline water is consumed and the PH level change is correct to what people have said, this can actually have a major positive effect on the body. It is a highly convenient way to help keep your PH level remain in range, but should not be used as the only solution. It should be used in moderation and in conjunction with the diet, with most of the Alkalizing effects coming from your food.

If you happen to be vegetarian or vegan, this diet can easily work for you as the food contents are nearly all vegetables and fruits.

The recipes included have not been written with using meats in mind, although one or two have meat or fish as the primary source of protein as they were written as a balanced meal which gives the 80/20 split of alkalizing/other foods as is recommended. So, if you read a recipe and meat or fish is included, you can just omit this and continue with the recipe as it is, or you can add something to substitute the meat or fish which could work just as well. Either way, you choose, because they are designed so they are highly adaptable and varied in tastes, so there is something there that will satisfy your appetite.

As with most other diets, it is advisable to seek a consultation with your trusted health professional, especially if you are on any current medication or have any ailments or illnesses. Although it is not the basis of this book - it is also a good recommendation to complete the recommended amount of daily exercise which is 30 minutes. This does not need not be anything over excessive, maybe just squats or stretches that you can do in your own home, and this you can split into 15 minute sessions one in the morning and one 15-minute session in the evening. It is also important to note if you are following this diet for weight loss, restrict the amount times that you weigh yourself to once or maybe twice per week, as your body fluctuates daily – and it could actually seem like you have gained weight instead of losing it, but that may not be the case. Stay positive every day too.

## Chapter 2: Alkaline Foods vs. Acidic Foods

Here I will explain the difference between Alkaline foods and Acidic foods, and how they interchange with each other. Firstly, foods being Acidic or Alkaline is not what you imagine, you would think a lemon is acidic just because of the bitter taste, but foods are termed Alkaline or Acidic depending what happens in your kidneys, essentially. So once the nutrients from the food reach your kidneys they produce either more ammonium which is classed as acidic, or they produce more bicarbonate which is classed as alkaline. Now scientists have created a way for this to be measured so foods can be measured and rated, and this score is called PRAL (Potential Renal Acid Load).

Example: Grains, Meat, Fish, and Eggs are considered acidic and have a positive PRAL score, on the other hand, fruits and vegetables are considered alkaline and have a negative PRAL score.

If you have too many acidic foods in your diet the main fear is you having bone loss, which occurs because your body takes minerals from your bones to optimize your body's whole PH level.

With this diet we aim for the 80/20 split. 80 percent alkaline, and 20 per cent 'other' foods that are not made up of processed foods or sugary foods. The 20 per cent would be meats, fish, poultry, eggs etc.

As with a lot of diets, the Alkaline diet consists of mainly fruits and vegetables -examples of the best are:

Raisins, dates, mushrooms, citrus fruits, tomatoes, spinach, celery, and cabbage to name but a few.

All raw foods are actually better than cooked; you should aim to eat a good percentage of your diet uncooked. As this has been said to be biogenic or life-giving. When you cook foods you actually reduce the minerals in them that help stabilize your alkalinity although, you still gain the normal vitamin advantage.

One really easy way to increase the amount of raw food intake is to juice, this way you can reduce the amounts of what you eat to just one or two glassfuls per day. This will also bombard your body with extra nutrients and vitamins due to the pure concentration. Legumes and nuts are other good choices, examples being almonds, green beans, lima beans and walnuts. Green drinks or supplements which are made from green vegetables and grasses in a powder form, these are loaded with many alkaline forming foods like chlorophyll - which has a structure very similar to human blood.

Acid foods or Anti-Alkaline foods are widely varied and constitute most of the average person's diet. Processed foods are one of the main culprits, as they contain high levels of sodium chloride (better known as table salt). Too much of this can lead to clogged arteries which restrict blood vessels and the creation of added acidity.

Let's take a look at Acid /Anti-Alkaline Foods:

Processed cereals e.g. cornflakes.

Milk, this creates high acidity in the body and contain carbohydrates, as do most calcium-rich dairy products. To counteract this, you should eat lots of leafy greens or juice using leafy greens e.g. kale, spinach etc.

Whole wheat products, it does not matter if they are whole or not, they all create acidity in the body. Surveys show Americans eat most of their plant food in the form of processed corn or wheat.

Eggs, lentils, soft drinks, and coffee are all high acidic foods. Peanuts, walnuts pasta, packaged grain, and bread are also all foods with a high acidic PRAL rating.

As well as the foods we eat, there are other things that can cause high acidity, alcohol and drug abuse (including prescription drugs), high caffeine intake, artificial sweeteners, stress and excess animal meats and hormones from foods. E.g. health and beauty products. Now although this list is not complete, it shows how exposure to many different things can lead to excessive acid build up within the human body.

If you feel like you have an unbalanced diet, or you have an illness where you have had no success from normal treatments, then maybe it is time to consider the Alkaline diet before any further long-term damage can be done. Due to an increased amount of Alkaline foods and minimal exposure to Acidic foods or anything that causes Acidic symptoms, you will start to feel the benefits even just after a short time. In most cases, not only will you be cancelling out the acidity in your body, you will be exposing your body to massive amounts of much-needed nutrients. This needs to be maintained as a lifestyle change, otherwise the acidic PH may cause unwanted symptoms, illness or decreased longevity. So, make the change for good, for the benefit of the long term.

# Chapter 3: The Health Benefits of an Alkaline Diet Long Term

After you have decided to change to the Alkaline diet and start your way on the road to a healthy lifestyle, or even if you have any ailments, then this will hopefully benefit your road to recovery. Many people may miss the meat aspect of the diet, but to balance it out you can follow the 80/20 rule, this is 80 percent Alkaline foods and 20 percent Acidic foods, which gives a good balance and enough Alkaline foods to keep your PH level in the perfect, healthy range.

As the Alkaline Diet is a long term strategy to get your body back in balance and keep it in range, there are many changes inside the body that we will not see, but we will still reap the benefits of. Exponentially, the longer you remain on the diet the more benefits you can achieve. Studies have been conducted and results show that diseases and illnesses are unable to survive in a body that is in an alkaline state. This theory has already had proven results which can possibly go on to achieve so much more. People have stated since they have gone onto greens, either by eating (or the more modern way, by juicing) have seen alleviations in skin problems, weight loss and even depression symptoms. Some used to have chronic hay fever but now use no medication, and some state their diabetes condition has been reversed and circulation in their outer limbs is much improved with hardly any swelling. More miraculously, some have made major statements stating the symptoms of cancer and heart disease have gone into reversal, and they have suffered no other ill effects.

Similar studies have shown over long periods, patients with back pain and muscle wasting have also seen improvements, these ailments are likely to be linked to the fact that once your body is in an acidic state, nutrients are leached from the bones over long periods.

Like most diets after a couple of days, there will be one or two short term side effects, these being headaches, tiredness, and mild dizziness, but these are normal and nothing to be alarmed about as they will quickly pass. From then you will start to feel the benefits once your body has been detoxed, and you will see an increase in energy levels, skin condition will improve and you will have a better mood too. The mood felt by you and your amount of concentration levels, will also noticeably increase.

It is safe to say the Alkaline diet is one of the best diets to be on, it is not a fad diet like many but it is a step back to how people used to eat in days gone by, when there was no industrialized food crop processing, no insecticides or pesticides to harm us, like in the modern world today. And eating a balanced diet of fruit and vegetables was just a natural way of life. Unfortunately, it is only recently our food crop processing has been industrialized and now we are starting to see the effects daily.

Every day we see reports of people becoming ill, becoming obese, being diagnosed with different illnesses etc., most of which is down to the average person's daily diet, with one of the main culprits being salt and long term acidity. Once you are on the Alkaline diet, the amount of processed salt will also be greatly reduced. So this will help clear your arteries and help the flow of blood around the body which takes the strain off the heart thus giving improved circulation. It is this improved blood flow that can now efficiently carry oxygen around the body and to the brain, for this reason, people with diabetes will see improvements (as they often suffer from bad circulation in their outer limbs).

Another group of people who are affected by acidosis is children, it has been found that they can have a shortage of the growth hormone, and this can be resolved by increasing the bicarbonate and potassium citrate levels. The 80/20 concept is needed as these increased levels will beneficially help their body start to increase the production of the growth hormone - which in turn helps the child to grow naturally and free from many illnesses and disease.

It has also been found postmenopausal women also have limited growth hormone development. So by increasing the potassium bicarbonate levels in these women, it can essentially lead them to an improved life, body posture and memory improvements.

If you have no major ailments, and you start the Alkaline diet just to feel healthy, or lose weight and get your body back in order, you will notice increased energy throughout the day. You can sleep better, it has also been said, sex is better. You will gain improved skin condition, your hair will feel in healthier, and your mood will be more positive. It is difficult to say what you will feel once you have been on the Alkaline diet long term if you have major ailments - as your body can take a lot more to get back on track due to the severity of the ailment. Hopefully improvements will occur quickly, and once you have started to overcome your ailments, you will start to feel the better skin, the better sleep etc.

As with a lot of diets which come and go, there are always bad points and downsides to using them long term, as the Alkaline diet is more of a way of life, and can be adapted to the 80/20 rule (which includes minimal acidic food intake) so as to allow you to gain the correct amount of natural fatty acids your body requires. To this effect, there are no major reports of the Alkaline diet not being suitable for the long term. Treat it as a lifestyle change, and know that this really is achievable through the 80/20 rule. You can look and feel fantastic, and also be allowed a treat here and there too. It is definitely a sustainable choice, for a better life through nutrition.

## Chapter 4: Scientific Merit

Dr. Otto Warburg was of German nationality and born in 1883, his father was a physicist and who probably gave Warburg the idea to go into medicine. Throughout his career, he was awarded many accolades for his studies into the assimilation of carbon dioxide in plants and how this was linked to tumors, including how oxygen is transferred. He is often thought of as the grandfather of the Alkaline Diet, as it was his discoveries that led the way for quite a few innovations in the medical field that are still be used and developed to this day.

After all his earlier accolades, his biggest achievement was winning the Nobel Peace Prize for his findings in a cure for cancer; all of this was in 1931 up until which he had been nominated a total of 46 times. His studies found cancer cells can only survive in an acidic state and also that they cannot survive in an oxygen rich environment, which is what your body would be, in a balanced PH state. This is one of the reasons the Alkaline diet is successful in the fight against cancers and other diseases, because once the host's body is an alkaline state, the cells that tend to cause cancer are unable to thrive. The cancer cells were found to be low on oxygen and had changed from using normal oxygen to survive, but were taking a more primitive form of respiration by utilizing sugars in the body. It was this discovery that led to new ways in the fields of cellular metabolism and how cells breathe. So it is important to notice the detrimental need to cut processed sugars from the diet, to aid in the 'non-cancer' formation process.

Dr. Warburg also thought most diseases were caused by pollution, as this leads the body to have over exposure to toxins. So when these toxins merge with cells that are undernourished, full of natural oxygen and hydrated by sugar – then this is the primary cause of cancer. When this happens, the cells build up an internal defense mechanism, they use sugar fermentation for producing oxygen, where they multiply and they refuse to die. It is the cancer cells themselves that turn a body into a highly Acidic state as cancer progresses.

It was Dr. Warburg's discoveries that found giving cells the clean oxygen they need can result in the cancer cells not being able to multiply, or at their best slowly beginning to die. This is where the Alkaline Diet comes into force, as your body will produce more oxygen in the blood, and the amount of fermented sugars cancer cells can feed on is dramatically reduced, and can sometimes be reversed.

Dr. Warburg was the author of many books and was a foreign member of the Royal Society of London. He was also made a Doctor honors at Oxford University.

Up until 1970 when Dr. Warburg died, he was still studying and researching, although now he was working part time with Dr. Carl Reich. Here they were completing final experiments regarding cancer, the results of which would have led to the publishing of a book with their findings which - would have changed the way cancer is treated completely. It is said that after his death, Dr. Reich was unable to collect his private equipment that was used in their experiments or any of the research they had done. It was also discovered that these discoveries had still not been released to the public.

Some of the later findings by Dr. Warburg were related to the lack of enzymes in cooked foods which causes red blood cells to cluster together. Once these foods have an enzyme deficiency they are unable to travel through smaller veins, and this causes circulation problems in different areas of the body. Additionally, it is in these parts of the body that have limited or no oxygen where cancer develops, but once you are in a stable alkaline state, there should be no reason for these areas to have built up blood cells, as the blood cells will be fully oxygenated and be able to flow freely.  Now you can see the importance of balancing your body PH level by introducing greens, legumes, and healthy doses of fruits into your diet. It is the aim to force the cells that would at one time use the sugars to feed, but will now have to revert to oxygen for breathing. If you have any ailments, illness or disease, (even ones that you don't know you have), these can be cured or put into reverse before they culminate with the non-oxygenated cells that can lead cancer to form. According to Warburg in clinical studies.

It is hard to believe the work of one man, for the most of his career has led the way to so many ideas and developments within the medical industry. In addition, if it was not for him it could have been another hundred years before anyone had linked the pieces together. On top of this, all the benefits of the Alkaline Diet and treatment of diseases that were thought to be incurable (or at least only treatable with drugs and chemotherapy) can be done with simplicity, by improving and maintaining your diet.

Most illnesses and diseases are not caused by mother nature; they are created by man. It is long-term exposure to highly processed products and toxins in our everyday lives that slowly but surely pushes our bodies out of balance, and into an unsafe Acidic state.

At the end of the day, everything you need to combat your illness or disease is a little help from mother nature and a little help from yourself. It is for this reason, I would like to thank Dr. Otto Warburg, even though he is not here to see what others have achieved, but he would be proud and happy for all the people he has been able to help. For your amazing contributions to the human cause, thank you Dr. Warburg, we salute you.

# Chapter 5: Blending Fruits and Vegetables to Make Them Superfoods

As the Alkaline diet is primarily all greens with little protein and dairy, it can be difficult for some people to adapt to, especially if faced with a very large serving of greens. Therefore, it is also advised to eat a percentage of your vegetable intake raw. With regards to this, there is a variation on the traditional Alkaline diet which is the 80/20 split, with the 80% being Alkaline foods and the 20% being proteins and treats that are not processed or full or processed sugars. This split should be enough for most people to get their PH levels back into shape and reap the benefits associated with it, as well.

The method for this is something you may have heard of called, "juicing" and this is where greens, fruits, and nuts are blended to such a degree that all the vital vitamins are released, and it is these drinks that can give maximum nutrition in an easy method without the need for eating massive meals. Although it is worth mentioning not all blenders and juicers are the same, a blender might not work at all, because it is not designed to break down foods to such as degree they can be drunk. On the other hand, juicers are designed to squash and twist the fruit - and in the process extracting all the juice. One drawback with these juicers is they leave the skins behind along with some other vegetable parts, and guess what it is in the skin? You guessed it, nutrients. Unfortunately, some are being thrown away when in fact they could be helping to boost your PH level significantly.

Recently, there have been a few machines released onto the market which improves on both the blender and juicer, with one of the most popular names being the "Nutri Bullet", which is the original nutrient extractor. This machine is able to break vegetables, fruits, and nuts down into a state that is most easily absorbed by the body. Every component of the food gets broken down, skins included to release the vitamins and minerals that you need. It is during this process that all seeds, nuts, and fibers are broken down into a liquid form that is easy to consume without any strenuous chewing. It also changes the molecular structure of the food, which can actually benefit the process by unlocking essential nutrients more easily.

There are many diets around that just make use of consuming juices for a period, and this can be hard for most people to adhere to as there is no physical chewing involved. With the Alkaline diet, you get the best of both worlds, eating at regular times and being able to super boost your body with one or two drinks throughout the day.

By adding green or natural fruit juicing to your regime, you will maximize the effects of the Alkaline diet and should see benefits that you did not think were possible, especially in such a short period of time. One thing that is worth mentioning, as the Alkaline diet recommends eating a part of your diet consisting of uncooked vegetables, this is the easiest way to make this happen. So you just choose your recipe, wash your veggies or fruit and whizz them into a 100 percent pure drink that not only tastes nice but is refreshing at the same time. With machines like this and all the health benefits you can obtain, it is easy to say why these drinks are truly classed as superfoods. Essentially, not will you only get all the nutrients and vitamins you require, but these green drinks will help flush toxins out of your system. Add honey to make them sweeter if needed.

### *Example Juice Drink:*

Serves 1

¾ cup cold coconut water

½ packed cup baby spinach

1/2 cup frozen berries

1 tbsp. flax seeds or chia seeds

½ cup kale

1/2 apple (cored)

1/2 cucumber

Small bunch mint leaves

¼ cup parsley leaves

½ handful mint leaves

1 lemon (juiced)

1-inch fresh ginger

Honey (to taste)

Now all you have to do is add all the ingredients to the Nutri Bullet or equivalent machine you may have. Just turn it on and let the machine do its magic, this should take about one minute or until the drink reaches a nice consistency.

This is just an example of one drink, but you can add, change or create your own flavors. It is possible for you to create juices which consist just of fruit - although some fruits contain natural sugars which are classed as acidic. Although still a healthy option, it is advised that greens and alkaline vegetables be used as much as possible. It has to be noted, carrots and coconut juice contain sugar but once consumed they have an alkalizing effect. So this is fine.

With all the benefits of the Alkaline diet and adding the juice delivery system into the mix, it is easy to see why nutritionists are now starting to pay more attention. They have realized when your body is in an acidic state it has to work twice as hard to bring your body into a safe PH range. This won't happen without any help from the individual acting on alkalinity. The acidity then takes the nutrients it needs from calcium reserves - and eventually the minerals from our bones. If this state continues undetected it can lead to some of the severe problems I have previously mentioned and much more serious consequences, including disease and/or cancer.

To summarize the whole principals of the Alkaline diet, a step that is required is to reduce your toxic load, is achieved by cutting out processed foods and replacing them with natural foods. As well as cutting out unhealthy acid forming foods, you have to supply fuel to your body with alkaline foods. The most cleansing alkaline foods which will help remove toxins are all leafy greens, green beans, legumes, almonds, hazelnuts, lemons, limes, figs and raisins. These can all be used in your normal diet and incorporated into your meals, or some can be adapted to be used in your juicing practices.

# Chapter 6: The Importance of Antioxidants and Alkaline Foods

Here I will explain more about the importance and roles the antioxidants play in foods, and the benefits of nutrients and vitamins on the body.

All foods consist of different mineral elements, amounts of nutrients and vitamins, and it is for this reason, we have to monitor and maintain a balanced diet to make sure we have enough of each. Above all, one of the most important contents of foods is the level of antioxidants which they contain, and some foods supply these in different amounts. How the foods are comprised determines how efficient they are at being released into the body.

Antioxidants at the most basic explanation work at a cellular level, to both repair and prevent oxidation from damage by free radicals. It is normal for people to have a small amount of free radical damage as this is part of the aging process, and so the body is built to cope with a certain amount of oxidation. However once oxidation starts to accelerate, this is where we start to have problems, because it limits the cells' ability to release acidic waste, which can be discarded through natural means. Additionally, this can lead to inflammation and also cause a drastic drop in the body's PH level.

There are many reasons that cause this rapid oxidation, the most poignant include: pollution, stress, pesticides, antibiotics, and preservatives. So to minimize free radical damage, it is very important to reduce exposure to as many free radicals as possible, or increase the quantity of antioxidant foods as much as possible to counteract the effects. As we all know the best source of antioxidants is in foods, with some of the top ones being: blackberries, strawberries, walnuts, spinach, kale amongst others.

You will be glad to hear that antioxidant-rich foods are also the alkalizing foods you will be eating - so you will have all the benefits and nutrition you expect and will have a limited buildup of uric acid, too. The Alkaline diet consisting of 80% Alkaline foods and 20 % Acidic foods is normally enough to repair damage and keep the levels in check. Positivity and stress reduction can also benefit individuals greatly.

One more function of antioxidants is to help the immune system function correctly, this alone is good enough reason to be eating antioxidant rich foods. There are many autoimmune illness sufferers that can be treated successfully with these additions.

There are many types of antioxidants, but you probably know them by other names. One great antioxidant is Vitamin E, and this antioxidant is a tremendous benefit for your heart, because it has the capacity to cleanse bad cholesterol from your arteries. This enables the blood to flow freely so reducing blockage that can build up from prolonged bad cholesterol - which leads to strokes and heart attacks. Antioxidants can also benefit diabetes sufferers as free radicals can easily thrive in the altered metabolic states of diabetics. With the correct type and number of antioxidants you can protect your blood vessels, kidneys, eyes and heart from harmful damage.

It is also the effects of free radicals that can cause cancer cells to grow, and there have been many studies that have linked the following cancer types to free radicals, including: colon, breast, prostate and stomach. Although it may not be possible for everyone to successfully prevent cancer, it will give you a fighting chance that you and everyone else deserves.

It is worth noting, you can buy antioxidants from health shops, although is it recommended to gain these from your leafy greens and not rely on pills.

I will now give a few examples of different fruits and vegetables and how they compare with vitamins and minerals. Black and green teas are full of antioxidants too. So drink them with limited additional sugar, for lasting, regular benefits.

### Vegetables

**Cucumber Minerals:** Potassium, Magnesium, Sodium, Calcium and Selenium, Vitamins: C, B1, B2, B6, A, K and E.

**Kale Minerals:** Potassium, Magnesium, Calcium, Iron and Selenium, Vitamins A, C, E, K, Pantothenic Acid, B1, B2 and B6.

**Tomato Minerals:** Potassium, Phosphorous, Magnesium, Calcium, Vitamins A, B1, B2, B6, C, K and E.

**Sweet Potato Minerals:** Potassium, Magnesium, Calcium, Manganese, Copper, Vitamins: C, B1, B2, B6, A, K and E.

## Fruits

**Banana Minerals:** Potassium, Magnesium, Calcium, Vitamins: A, B1, B2, B6, C, E and K.

**Blackberries:** Minerals Potassium, Magnesium, Calcium, Sodium Vitamins: A, B1, B2, B3, C, E and K.

Dates Minerals: Potassium, Phosphorous, Magnesium, Calcium, Vitamins: A, B1, B2, B6, Niacin and Vitamin E

## Nuts and Seeds and Rice and Wheat

**Almonds Minerals:** Potassium, Calcium, Magnesium, Vitamins: B1, B2, B6, E.

**Coconut Minerals:** Potassium, Calcium, Magnesium, Vitamins C, B1, B2, Folate, E.

**Sunflower Seeds Minerals**: Potassium, Calcium, Magnesium, Vitamins Niacin, Folate, A, K and E.

**Brown Rice Minerals:** Potassium, Calcium, Magnesium, Vitamins, B1, B2, Niacin and folate.

***Hard Red Wheat Minerals:*** Potassium, Phosphorous, Magnesium, Sodium, Vitamins: Niacin, A, E and K.

As you can see, the amount of goodness that is in foods includes minerals and nutrients. The above is not a complete list - these are just the main ones, for each type of food. Also, the levels of the minerals and vitamins can alter quite a lot, this is why we need to check which foods give the most benefit for the Alkaline diet and which ones we can use that gives us a wide variety of choice.

When it comes around to do your grocery shopping, you should try to buy organic if possible, as they are grown more naturally than mass industrialized food crops, and they can contain up to thirty percent more nutrients as they are not exposed to pesticides etc.

Above, I have only spoken about Alkaline foods and the nutrient and vitamin benefit, this does not include any proteins or meats, so if you stick to the recommendations of 20% acidic foods, the 80% of alkaline food types that I have mentioned, that will work well. I will gladly get you on track to becoming healthy and feeling amazing again. If you have any ailments, there is a chance you will be amazed when they start to vanish or lessen. Sometimes you may not even notice they have gone, just that you do not have the symptoms or aches anymore. So we can certainly aim for that.

# Chapter 7: Breakfasts

### Muesli Mix with Berries

Serves 2

2 cups of unsweetened almond milk (plain or flavored)

½ cup of raw almonds

½ cup of raw pumpkin seeds

¼ cup walnuts

2 tbsp. of chia seeds

2 tbsp. of flaxseeds

Cinnamon to taste

Honey to taste

¼ cup berries of choice

### Instructions

In a medium bowl add all of the ingredients except the cinnamon and the honey, mix well until combined.

Cover and store in refrigerator overnight.

Remove from refrigerator divide between two bowls.

Add berries of choice and top with cinnamon and honey.

## Tofu Scramble

Serves 2

½ white onion diced

1 cup extra firm tofu

1 clove of garlic minced

2 tsp. coconut oil

1 tsp. smoked paprika

1/2 tsp. turmeric

1 tsp dried parsley (or fresh if you have some)

2 cup baby kale or spinach leaves (roughly chopped)

2 large tomatoes

1 medium avocado

## Instructions

Peel and remove seed on avocado and cut into slices.

By hand crumble the tofu until you have medium sized pieces.

Cut tomatoes in half and cook under the heated grill or cook in a skillet with a little oil.

Heat a skillet over medium high heat and sauté the onion and garlic in the coconut oil until soft.

Add spices and tofu and cook until tofu is cooked through and starting to brown.

Add kale and spinach leaves and cook until tender.

Divide tofu mixture, tomatoes and avocado between two serving plates.

## Pancakes

Serves 4

2 cup whole meal spelt flour

½ cup sesame seeds

1/2 cup pumpkin seeds

1/2 cup flax seeds

1 cup chia seeds

3 tsp. of baking soda

1 tsp sea salt

Large pinch of stevia

Unsweetened almond milk

Coconut oil for frying

### Instructions

Place all seeds in food processor and grind into a flour (divide into 2 and use one-half, save another half for next time).

In large bowl combine seed flour with whole meal spelt flour.

Add baking soda and salt and the stevia.

Add almond milk slowly while mixing until you have a creamy consistency batter.

Preheat a nonstick pan and add a small amount of coconut oil.

Pour 1 ladle of mixture into pan and cook on medium heat until bubbles start to form on the top then flip and cook until golden.

Serve warm with lemon juice and honey.

## *Berries and Quinoa Porridge*

Serves 2

1 cup berries of choice

½ tsp stevia

½ tsp cinnamon

½ cup water

1 ½ cup almond milk plain or vanilla flavor

2 tbsp. chia seeds soaked overnight

½ cup quinoa

1 tsp vanilla (optional)

## *Instructions*

Heat a saucepan over medium heat and add quinoa, season with cinnamon and cook while stirring until toasted about 3 minutes.

Add the almond milk, water and vanilla and stir in the stevia and salt.

Bring to a low boil, then lower the heat and cook until the grains are tender, if the liquid has dried, add more water and cook for about 25 minutes, stir frequently to prevent burning.

Divide into serving bowls and add berries of choice.

### Chia Pudding with Seasonal Fruits and Nuts

Serves 2

56 g chia seeds

6 almonds (finely chopped for topping)

½ tsp vanilla

½ tsp cinnamon

2 cups almond milk (plain or vanilla unsweetened)

Stevia to taste

1 cup seasonal fruits for topping

### Instructions

Combine all chia seeds, vanilla, cinnamon, almond milk into a large container mix well and store covered in refrigerator overnight.

Remove from refrigerator add stevia to taste and mix well.

Divide between two bowls and top with fruits and chopped nuts.

### Raisin and Date Quinoa

Serves 2

½ cup quinoa

4 pitted dates

2 tbsp. raisins

Cinnamon

### Instructions

Cook the quinoa as per packet instructions, bring to a boil then simmer for about 15 minutes.

Chop dates into small pieces and add to quinoa with raisins.

Divide between 2 bowls and sprinkle with cinnamon.

Serve warm.

### Chilled Oats with Yogurt and Fruit

Serves 2

1 cup of berries or fruits

1 cup yogurt

1 cup skimmed milk

1 cup of oats

1 tbsp. peanut butter

1 tsp cinnamon

1 banana

### Instructions

Divide first five ingredients between 2 sealable glass jars, seal and place in refrigerator overnight.

Remove from refrigerator and add banana slices and cinnamon.

## Millet Porridge with Maple Syrup and Raisins

½ cup of millet

A pinch of salt

½ tbsp. cinnamon

¼ cup of maple syrup

5 cups of water

### Instructions

In a large saucepan add water and bring water to a boil.

Add salt and millet, cover and reduce heat then simmer for 15 minutes.

Add cinnamon and cook for 20 minutes.

Add maple syrup, raisins and stir.

Cook until desired thickness has been reached.

Divide between serving bowls and eat warm.

### Nut Cream with Fresh Fruits

Serves 2

250g macadamia nuts

80g almonds

2 cup almond milk

1 tbsp. vanilla powder

1 tsp stevia

500g mixed berries

### Instructions

Soak macadamia and almonds overnight.

Drain and add to blender, add all other ingredients excluding berries.

Blend until you have a smooth creamy texture.

Chill in freezer until firm then serve with fresh berries.

# Chapter 8: Lunches

## Spicy Tofu Wraps

Serves 2

4 whole wheat tortillas

½ packet of firm tofu

1 avocado diced

1/8 cup toasted almonds

4 large lettuce leaves

1 bell pepper (sliced thinly)

2 celery stalks (sliced thinly)

1 medium onion (sliced thinly)

1 large tomatoes (sliced thinly)

2 tbsp. chili sauce

### Instructions

Crumble tofu into a small bowl and mix with chili sauce.

Warm tortillas in a dry skillet.

Place lettuce leaf on each tortilla.

Place tofu and chili sauce mix.

Add vegetable strips and chopped nuts.

### *Hearty Broccoli Broth*

Serves 2

4 cups vegetable stock

2 green onions (chopped)

1 red bell pepper (chopped)

2 celery stalks (chopped)

4 cups broccoli (chopped)

Salt to taste

Pepper to taste

2 cloves garlic minced

1-inch ginger (peeled and chopped finely)

### *Instructions*

In large saucepan bring stock to a boil then reduce heat, add broccoli, onions, bell pepper, minced garlic, ginger and celery cook for 5 minutes.

Place all ingredients in a blender and pulse for 2 minutes, add water if consistency is too thick.

Return to the pan to rewarm, add salt and pepper to taste.

Divide between serving dishes and serve warm.

### Asian Veggie Wraps

Serves 2

2 cups vegetable broth

1 medium onion (sliced thinly)

1 tsp cilantro (chopped finely)

½ cup bean sprouts

½ cup water chestnuts (sliced thinly)

1 red bell pepper (sliced into thin strips)

### Instructions

Scald cabbage leaves with hot water and leave in pan for 30 minutes.

Finely slice vegetables.

Lay vegetable strips into each cabbage leaf and sprinkle with chopped cilantro.

Roll leaf tight and fold in edges, use a toothpick to hold them closed.

Simmer in vegetable broth for 30 minutes or until tender.

Season with olive oil and cayenne pepper.

### *Mexican stuffed Tofu Pita*

Serves 2

4 whole wheat pita bread

3 cloves garlic (minced)

2 medium chilies (finely chopped)

1 pack firm tofu

1 tsp Mexican seasoning

¼ cup onion (minced)

1 tbsp. cilantro (finely chopped)

1 jar enchilada sauce

¼ cup soy parmesan cheese substitute

### *Instructions*

Toast pita bread and cut in half.

In a medium bowl crumble tofu until you have large crumbs mix in Mexican seasoning.

Add minced garlic, onion, and chili to a skillet and sauté until tender, add tofu and cook until start to brown all over.

Open each pita pocket and place a couple of spoonsful of mixture inside.

When hot, pour enchilada sauce inside pocket then sprinkle with parmesan cheese substitute.

### Onion Stew with Tofu

Serves 2

3 cloves garlic

2 medium onions (sliced)

2 large onions (diced)

1 pack tofu

4 kale leaves (torn)

2 cabbage leaves (torn)

1 bay leaf

2 cups green beans

Salt & pepper (to taste)

3 cups of water

Coconut oil (for frying)

### Instructions

Steam fry the sliced onions in a pan with lid.

Add water bay leaf, kale and cabbage simmer until soft.

Remove bay leaf and add diced onions and green beans, simmer until beans are tender.

Cut tofu into small chunks, add oil to skillet and fry until golden brown.

Divide onion stew between dishes and top with warm tofu.

Add salt & pepper to taste.

### Crunchy Spinach and Rocket Salad

Serves 2

250 g fresh spinach

250 g fresh rocket

2 tbsp. lemon juice

Stevia to taste

1 large avocado (diced)

¼ cup walnuts

¼ cup almonds

Braggs liquid aminos (to taste)

¼ cup olive oil

1 clove garlic (minced)

### Instructions

Wash and trim spinach and rocket then pat dry.

Chop almonds and walnuts and toast in dry skillet.

In a large bowl add olive oil, garlic, amino acids, stevia and lemon juice.

Add avocado spinach and rocket, toss well to coat everything.

Divide between plates and top with chopped nuts.

### *Avocado Salad with Toasted Almonds*

Serves 4

1 head of lettuce (any variety of choice)

1 packet of baby spinach

2 medium tomatoes (cut into wedges)

¼ cup pitted olives (sliced)

2 large avocado (diced)

1 medium green pepper (de-seeded and thinly sliced)

1 medium red pepper (de-seeded and thinly sliced)

1 medium cucumber (sliced)

½ cup chopped almonds

### *Salad Dressing*

1 tbsp. olive oil

3 tbsp. lemon juice

½ tsp finely chopped oregano

½ tsp finely chopped cilantro

¼ tsp black pepper

¼ tsp cayenne pepper

## Instructions

Prepare dressing – in a small jar combine lemon juice, olive oil, oregano, cilantro, cayenne pepper, and pepper and shake well.

Wash and dry lettuce leaves and baby spinach and place in salad bowl.

Add bell peppers, tomatoes, avocado, olives and cucumber then pour over the dressing. Gently toss to coat everything.

Chop almonds and lightly roast in a dry skillet.

Divide between serving plates and top with roasted nuts.

### Soup with Lentils

Serves 2

125 g lentils

1 carrot thinly (sliced)

1 leek thinly (sliced)

1 onion (diced)

4 cloves of garlic (minced)

2 tbsp. olive oil

1 tbsp. lemon juice

1 bay leaf

½ tsp oregano (finely chopped)

2 large tomatoes (chopped and crushed)

Salt and pepper (to taste)

4 cups of vegetable stock

### Instructions

Soak lentils overnight then rinse and drain.

In a large saucepan add enough water to cover lentils then cook as per packet instructions or until soft.

In a large saucepan add the vegetable stock, carrot, leek, onion, garlic and tomatoes and bring to a boil.

Add lentils and then partially cover and simmer for 1 hour, add more water if needed.

Add olive oil and lemon juice then season if required.

Divide between serving dishes, serve hot.

## Zingy Quinoa Bowls with Rocket

Serves 2

¼ cup cooked quinoa

1 avocado

¼ cup chopped almonds

¼ cup apple cider vinegar

¼ cup olive oil

3 tbsp. lemon juice

Zest of half lemon

½ tsp salt

Pepper (to taste)

1/2 tsp chili flakes

¼ cup pine nuts

4 cups chopped rocket

### Instructions

Mix olive oil, apple cider vinegar, lemon juice, lemon zest and chili flakes.

In a large bowl add rocket and top with diced avocado, pine nuts, almonds and quinoa.

Pour dressing on top and toss to combine.

Salt and pepper to taste.

## Grilled Avocado and Olives

Serves 2

2 large avocados

3 tbsp. lemon juice

Olive oil

2 medium tomatoes chopped

8 olives chopped

### Instructions

Heat griddle pan on medium high heat.

Cut avocado in half and brush with olive oil and lemon juice.

Place face down and cook until grill marks appear about 3 to 4 minutes.

Add spoonful of chopped olives and tomato to each avocado half.

Season lightly with salt and pepper if required.

# Chapter 9: Main Meals

## *Veggie Curry*

Serves 2

800 ml coconut milk

100 ml vegetable stock

500 g assorted vegetables (carrots, broccoli, cauliflower, green beans)

6 large mushrooms

3 bay leaves

1 shallot

8 garlic cloves (chopped)

2 lemongrass stalks

½ tsp black pepper

3 tbsp. curry powder

2-inch chopped ginger

½ tsp salt

5 chili chopped

1 tbsp. turmeric powder

Olive oil

250 g fish fillet or chicken breast optional

## Instructions

In large pan place olive oil and sauté garlic, ginger, chili and shallot till soft.

Add vegetables and vegetable stock and cook for 10 minutes then add bay leaf, curry powder, turmeric, and lemongrass.

Add coconut milk and simmer for 20 minutes until vegetables are soft.

Towards the end of cooking time add mushrooms then taste and season with salt and pepper as required.

Serve with brown rice.

## Bag Steamed Fish

Serves 2

2 x 180 g white fish filet

3 tsp olive oil

1 lemon (zested and juiced)

1-inch ginger (minced)

2 garlic cloves (minced)

Salt

## Instructions

Preheat oven to 200 degrees Celsius.

Lay 2 pieces of tin foil on bench and lay fish fillet on each, cut 2 or 3 slits into top of each fish.

Spoon a small olive oil over each fish and then season with a little salt.

Place half of lemon zest and juice onto fish then place half of the ginger and garlic onto the fish.

Fold edges of foil to make a sealed packet.

Place onto a baking tray.

Baked for approximately 15 minutes or until done, depending on thickness of fish.

Remove from foil and serve hot with salad or steamed vegetables.

## Spaghetti Bolognese

Serves 2

200 g goats cheese

2 onions (chopped)

500 grams of soaked vegetable protein

2 carrots diced small

2 sticks of celery diced small

2 kg chopped tomatoes

3 tbsp. unsweetened tomato paste

Salt and pepper (to taste)

Vegan parmesan cheese

2 cloves of garlic

2 tbsp. olive oil

### Instructions

In large skillet add oil and sauté garlic and onions until soft add vegetable protein and cook until starting to brown, add tomatoes, celery, carrots and tomato paste, simmer for 1 hour.

Add water if sauce becomes too thick.

Cook whole wheat spaghetti as per packet instructions.

Divide pasta between plates and them serve half of the sauce mixture to the top.

### Veggie Lasagna

Serves 4

500 g zucchini

500 g eggplant

1/2 kg sweet potato

2 red bell peppers

1/2 cup unsweetened tomato sauce

150 g baby spinach leaves

30 g parmesan cheese substitute

### Instructions

Preheat oven to 180 degrees Celsius.

Slice zucchini into thin slices, then lay flat onto parchment paper lined baking tray and roast for 10 minutes, remove and set on one side.

Slice eggplant into short strips and place in a single layer on a baking tray and lightly brush with olive oil and season with a little salt and then roast for 30 minutes or until golden and soft.

Remove and set aside.

Thinly slice the sweet potato lengthways brush with olive oil and bake for 30 minutes.

Cut bell pepper in half and remove seeds, with skin facing up roast in oven for 20 – 30 minutes until soft then place in sealed plastic bag, after 30 minutes remove from plastic and peel skin.

In baking dish, spread thin layer of tomato sauce and cover with 1/3 of the sweet potato.

Top with half of the zucchini and top with a few baby spinach leaves, cover with eggplant and spread over tomato sauce, top with all the roasted bell peppers.

Repeat process with sweet potato, zucchini, spinach, eggplant and tomato.

For the top use the remaining third of sweet potato and cover with tomato sauce.

Top with crumbled goats cheese and parmesan alternative.

Place in hot oven and bake for 45 minutes.

Serve with salad (optional).

### Roast Chicken and Vegetables

200 grams of chicken breast (skinless)

6 large tomatoes (halved)

2 medium onions (cut into quarters)

4 celery stalks (cut into chunks)

¼ cup black olives

4 tbsp. olive oil

1 large zucchini (sliced)

2 red peppers (de-seeded and cut in quarters)

Salt and pepper (to taste)

1 large tbsp. pesto

### Instructions

Preheat oven to 350 degrees F.

Lay all the vegetables in a flat baking dish the sprinkle over the olives.

Make cuts crossways in the chicken breasts and lay on top of the vegetables.

Mix olive oil and pesto and spoon onto the chicken breasts.

Cover with foil and bake for 30 minutes.

Remove foil and cook for another 10 minutes until chicken is tender.

### *Peppered Tomato Pasta*

Serves 2

250g spelt pasta

150g tomatoes

1/4 cup sun dried tomatoes (chopped)

1 small red bell pepper (diced)

1 small zucchini (diced)

1 onion (diced)

2 garlic cloves (minced)

1 tsp chili flakes

5 basil leaves (finely chopped)

2-3 tbsp. olive oil

Salt and (pepper to taste)

### *Instructions*

Cook pasta as per packet instructions.

Dice all vegetables and finely chop onion and garlic.

In large skillet, heat oil and sauté the onion, garlic, chili flakes and bell pepper until soft.

Add tomatoes and zucchini and cook for another 10 minutes stirring occasionally.

Add basil and season with salt and pepper as necessary.

Divide warm pasta between serving plates and spoon tomato sauce on top of pasta.

### *Brown Rice and Stir Fry Veggies*

Serves 2

2 cups of wild rice

1/2 cup of pak choi

1/4 cup of broccoli

¼ cup cauliflower

1 cup green beans

2 cloves garlic (minced)

1 large carrot

1 cup bean sprouts

1 chili (chopped)

juice of 1 lemon

Cilantro (chopped)

Salt (to taste)

Basil

Olive oil

### *Instructions*

Cook rice as per packet instructions.

Chop all your vegetables and place in hot skillet with a little of oil, and cook until becoming tender.

In a pestle and mortar smash the chili and cilantro, add lemon juice and olive oil, mix well.

Divide rice between serving plates, top with vegetables and drizzle sauce on top.

### Crispy Pan Fried Tofu

Serves 2

2 pieces' firm tofu (you can change for 2 x 100 g fish fillet or 2 x 100 g chicken breast)

¼ cup ground almonds

4 tbsp. olive oil

Lemon juice of 1 lemon

½ tsp salt

1/4 tsp. pepper

¼ tsp cayenne pepper

### Instructions

Slice tofu pieces in half making two thin steak pieces.

In a bowl put ground almonds, salt, pepper and cayenne pepper and mix well.

For each steak soak in lemon juice then roll in nut mixture.

In a skillet put 2 tbsp. of oil and pan fry until crispy.

Serve with green salad.

## Leek Stir Fry

Serves 4

4 leek stalks (sliced)

2 cloves of garlic

3 medium onions (diced)

2 zucchinis (halved then sliced lengthways)

3 tomatoes (diced)

4 tbsp. olive oil

1 tsp salt

1 tsp oregano

1 tbsp. parsley

½ tsp curry powder

½ tsp turmeric

1 pinch black pepper

½ cup water

## Instructions

Heat oil in a skillet and sauté onions and garlic until soft and slightly brown.

Add leeks and zucchini and cook for 4 minutes while stirring.

Add water cover pan and simmer for about 10 minutes then add tomatoes, curry powder, turmeric and simmer covered for another 10 minutes.

Just before the end of the cooking season as necessary with salt and parsley.

Serve hot.

## Deli Dish

Serves 2

½ cup of almonds (soaked overnight)

½ tsp garam masala

2 cups of water

Pinch of salt

1 cup uncooked quinoa

¼ cups of raisins

½ tsp turmeric

½ tsp coriander

½ tsp cumin

## Instructions

Chop almonds and put on one side.

In medium pan add 2 cups of water and pinch of salt, add the quinoa and all the ingredients and stir to mix, lower heat and cover then simmer until quinoa is cooked and absorbed all the water.

Remove from heat and stand for 10 minutes, mix with a fork to fluff up, with fork mix in chopped almonds.

Divide between 2 plates and serve with green salad.

# Bonus Chapter: Alkalizing Drinks and Shakes

## Zinger

Serves 1

½ cucumber

½ avocado

1 handful kale or baby spinach

2 peeled limes

6 ice cubes

Stevia to taste

### Instructions

Add all ingredients to Nutri Bullet or equivalent machine (blender can work if needed).

Blend on high until you have a smooth consistency.

Pour into glass and drink immediately.

## Super Detox Shake

Serves 1

½ cup chopped celery

1 pear (cored and chopped)

1 banana (best frozen)

1 cup coconut water

½ lemon peeled

½ tbsp. chia seeds

½ inch ginger (peeled)

½ cucumber (chopped)

1 cup kale or spinach

1 cup romaine leaves

¼ cup almonds

Pinch of cinnamon

4 ice cubes

### Instructions

Place ingredients in Nutri Bullet or equivalent machine.

Blend until you have a smooth mixture.

Pour into a glass and drink immediately.

### Fruit with a Punch

1 mango

½ cup pineapple

2 cups kale or spinach

½ inch ginger

1 cup coconut water

4 ice cubes

### Instructions

Add ingredients to Nutri Bullet.

Blend until you have a smooth mixture.

Drink immediately.

## Strawberry Smoothie

1 cup of strawberries

1 ½ cups coconut water

2 tbsp. chia seeds

4 ice cubes

2 handfuls of kale or spinach

## Instructions

Add ingredients to Nutri Bullet.

Blend until you have a smooth mixture.

Drink immediately.

### Berry Blend

1 cup of blueberries (any berries can be used)

½ cup of almond yogurt

1 cup of almond milk

2 tablespoons of chia seeds

2 tbsp. flax seeds

### Instructions

Add ingredients to Nutri bullet.

Blend until you have a smooth mixture.

Drink immediately.

# Conclusion

I would like to thank you for buying this book it has been quite an experience. I feel that it makes all the difference if you write from experience and not just researching information. Also, from personal experience I feel like I can give a helping hand to those who need understanding, and are not just presented with pages of information. I would like once again to thank Dr. Warburg for his foresight into what we now know, it is from people who have helped people like me, who I hope can in turn also help you. Feel free to look up added information as required.

I have tried to give you just enough information on the things you need to know that will enable you to make the jump...and head down that road to good health and recovery. The recipes are just a glimpse of what is available and can quite easily be adapted to your own tastes, too. Additionally, I have mentioned it is not a diet, it is a new lifestyle. I do not want to tell you, "You must do this and must not do that," that is not how the Alkaline diet works, but what it does do is gives you the tools to be able to make your own choices. The choices that you will make an exceptional benefit from, and the glory belongs to you.

Please remember the 80/20 rule for success, as this can enable you to keep going without failure. You can still eat a few treats here and there, and enjoy a few hot cups of coffee. Good luck and best wishes, you've got this in the bag! Go you!